NNAAP
PRACTICE

National Nurse Aid
Assessment Program
Practice Questions

Published by

Complete TEST Preparation Inc.

Copyright © 2011 Complete Test Preparation Inc. ALL RIGHTS RESERVED. No part of this book may be reproduced or transferred in any form or by any means, graphic, electronic, or mechanical, including photocopying, recording, web distribution, taping, or by any information storage retrieval system, without the written permission of the author.

Notice: Complete Test Preparation Inc. makes every reasonable effort to obtain from reliable sources accurate, complete, and timely information about the tests covered in this book. Nevertheless, changes can be made in the tests or the administration of the tests at any time and Complete Test Preparation Inc. makes no representation or warranty, either expressed or implied as to the accuracy, timeliness, or completeness of the information contained in this book. Complete Test Preparation Inc. make no representations or warranties of any kind, express or implied, about the completeness, accuracy, reliability, suitability or availability with respect to the information contained in this document for any purpose. Any reliance you place on such information is therefore strictly at your own risk.

The author(s) shall not be liable for any loss incurred as a consequence of the use and application, directly or indirectly, of any information presented in this work. Sold with the understanding, the author is not engaged in rendering professional services or advice. If advice or expert assistance is required, the services of a competent professional should be sought.

The company, product and service names used in this publication are for identification purposes only. All trademarks and registered trademarks are the property of their respective owners. Complete Test Preparation Inc. is not affiliated with any educational institution.

We strongly recommend that students check with exam providers for up-to-date information regarding test content.

ISBN-13: 9781772452105

Version 6.2 January 2015

Published by
Complete Test Preparation Inc.
Canada
Visit us on the web at http://www.test-preparation.ca
Printed in the USA

About Complete Test Preparation

The Complete Test Preparation Team has been publishing high quality study materials since 2005. Thousands of students visit our websites every year, and thousands of students, teachers and parents all over the world have purchased our teaching materials, curriculum, study guides and practice tests.

Complete Test Preparation Inc. is committed to providing students with the best study materials and practice tests available on the market. Members of our team combine years of teaching experience, with experienced writers and editors, all with advanced degrees (Masters or higher).

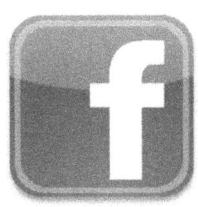

Find us on Facebook

www.facebook.com/CompleteTestPreparation

Contents

6 Getting Started

7 Practice Test Questions Set
        Quick Reference Answer Key   26
        Answer Key with Explanations   27

36 Practice Test Questions Set 2
        Quick Reference Answer Key   54
        Answer Key with Explanations   55

64 Conclusion

65 Multiple Choice Secrets Special Offer

Getting Started

CONGRATULATIONS! By deciding to take the National Nurse Aid Assessment Program (NNAAP), you have taken the first step toward a great future! Of course, there is no point in taking this important examination unless you intend to do your very best in order to earn the highest grade you possibly can. That means getting yourself organized and discovering the best approaches, methods and strategies to master the material. Yes, that will require real effort and dedication on your part but if you are willing to focus your energy and devote the study time necessary, before you know it you will be opening that letter of acceptance for the job of your dreams.

We know that taking on a new endeavour can be a little scary, and it is easy to feel unsure of where to begin. That's where we come in. This study guide is designed to help you improve your test-taking skills, show you a few tricks of the trade and increase both your competency and confidence.

The National Nurse Aid Assessment Program

While we seek to make our guide as comprehensive as possible, it is important to note that like all exams, the CNA Exam might be adjusted at some future point. New material might be added, or content that is no longer relevant or applicable might be removed. It is always a good idea to give the materials you receive when you register to take the CNA a careful review.

Practice Test 1

The practice test questions present questions that are representative of the type of question you should expect to find on the NNAAP. However, they are not intended to match exactly what is on the NNAAP.

For the best results, take this Practice Test as if it were the real exam. Set aside time when you will not be disturbed, and a location that is quiet and free of distractions. Read the instructions carefully, read each question carefully, and answer to the best of your ability.

Use the bubble answer sheets provided. When you have completed the Practice Test, check your answer against the Answer Key and read the explanation provided.

Remember – the purpose of a practice test is to learn! After completing the first practice test, mark your answers, then go back and review the explanations to see where you went wrong.

Answer Sheet – Practice Test I

	A	B	C	D	E		A	B	C	D	E
1	○	○	○	○	○	26	○	○	○	○	○
2	○	○	○	○	○	27	○	○	○	○	○
3	○	○	○	○	○	28	○	○	○	○	○
4	○	○	○	○	○	29	○	○	○	○	○
5	○	○	○	○	○	30	○	○	○	○	○
6	○	○	○	○	○	31	○	○	○	○	○
7	○	○	○	○	○	32	○	○	○	○	○
8	○	○	○	○	○	33	○	○	○	○	○
9	○	○	○	○	○	34	○	○	○	○	○
10	○	○	○	○	○	35	○	○	○	○	○
11	○	○	○	○	○	36	○	○	○	○	○
12	○	○	○	○	○	37	○	○	○	○	○
13	○	○	○	○	○	38	○	○	○	○	○
14	○	○	○	○	○	39	○	○	○	○	○
15	○	○	○	○	○	40	○	○	○	○	○
16	○	○	○	○	○	41	○	○	○	○	○
17	○	○	○	○	○	42	○	○	○	○	○
18	○	○	○	○	○	43	○	○	○	○	○
19	○	○	○	○	○	44	○	○	○	○	○
20	○	○	○	○	○	45	○	○	○	○	○
21	○	○	○	○	○	46	○	○	○	○	○
22	○	○	○	○	○	47	○	○	○	○	○
23	○	○	○	○	○	48	○	○	○	○	○
24	○	○	○	○	○	49	○	○	○	○	○
25	○	○	○	○	○	50	○	○	○	○	○

Case 1

Your supervisor has assigned you a patient, John, a 78-year-old man with Dementia. He fell out of his bed and sprained his wrist. He is diabetic and suffers from left-sided weakness due to a stroke. He requires total care and assistance with everything he does. He has dentures. He can no longer walk alone, feed himself, bathe or dress himself, and he is incontinent of urine and stool. His vital signs are to be monitored q 4 hrs.

1. You are preparing to shave John. You need to assemble your supplies. What is the first action that you should take?

    a. Place a warm damp towel around his face to soften his beard and relax him

    b. Check the chart to see if you should shave him and if so what type of razor you can safely use.

    c. Gather your towels, razor and shaving cream and proceed to John's room

    d. Make certain John has the privacy required to perform ADL's

2. You have checked the chart and it is safe to shave John using a standard razor. You should

    a. Draw the razor in the direction of hair growth

    b. Draw the razor opposite the direction of hair growth

    c. Pull the skin taut

    d. Both a and c

3. In performing John's daily care, you note that his toenails need to be trimmed. You should do which of the following?

    a. Gather your supplies and carefully trim his nails after cleaning his feet.
    b. Ignore it
    c. Note it in your documentation so that a doctor can cut his nails
    d. Plan to trim his nails while you are bathing him

4. When should you clean John's dentures?

    a. Before performing mouth care or cleaning
    b. After performing mouth care or cleaning
    c. Every 2 hours
    d. Before and after each meal

5. Oral care of any type should be performed

    a. At least twice per day
    b. After each meal
    c. Before and after each meal
    d. After each meal, in the morning and each night before the patient goes to sleep

6. To make John's bed, which of the following will you need?

    a. Gloves
    b. Clean linens, gloves, and a bag for dirty linens
    c. Clean linens and a bag for dirty linens
    d. Clean linens

7. When removing your contaminated gloves after making John's bed, you would

    a. Grasp the fingers of one glove using the other gloved hand and remove it

    b. Grasp the cuff of one gloved had using the other gloved hand and remove it

    c. Grasp the palm of one gloved hand using the other gloved hand and remove the glove leaving it in your remaining gloved hand. Then you would place your un-gloved fingers beneath the cuff of the remaining dirty glove, removing it by turning it inside out keeping the glove you have already removed inside the palm of the glove you are removing

    d. Grasp the fingers of each glove and remove them by gently tugging at the ends and dispose of them in the appropriate receptacle

8. John has gone down to radiology for a chest x-ray. You decide to take advantage of the time to make his bed. The first thing that you would do is

    a. Strip the bed of dirty linens

    b. Clear the room of visitors

    c. Roll the dirty linens into a ball, carry them held away from your body and deposit them in the dirty linen bag

    d. Maneuver the bed into its 'flat' position

9. The second thing that you should do in preparing to make John's bed is to

    a. Raise the bed to a comfortable working height

    b. Remove the dirty linens

    c. Gather your clean linens and other supplies

    d. None of the above

10. When removing the dirty linens from John's bed you would do which of the following?

    a.   You should just pull them off and carry them to the dirty linen bag and place them there

    b.   Loosen them and roll each end toward the center and carry them to the dirty linen bag

    c.   Remove each item individually and inspect it for blood and then take it to the dirty laundry bag

    d.   It doesn't matter how you remove the linens as long as they are placed in the appropriate receptacle

11. After removing the dirty linens, you notice that John's mattress is soiled. You should

    a.   Call and have the mattress replaced

    b.   Document your findings

    c.   Wipe the mattress down

    d.   Make the bed and have it ready for John

12. When preparing to make John's bed, you notice that his glasses are on the bed. You should (Choose the MOST correct answer)

    a.   Remove them while making the bed and place them on the bedside table

    b.   Document your findings

    c.   Put them in your pocket so that they will not get broken

    d.   All of the above

13. **The following day, you are once again assigned to be John's caregiver. You are preparing to make his bed, but he cannot get up today. You must make the bed with him in it. It is best, when making an occupied bed if**

    a. You can obtain assistance from a co-worker
    b. You get assistance from a family member
    c. Raise John's head to a 30 degree angle
    d. Document that you need to make the bed while John is in it

14. **John should be bathed**

    a. Daily
    b. Twice daily
    c. Only as needed
    d. None of the above

15. **To bathe John, you will need**

    a. Towels, three sheets, bath cloths, soap, warm water and a basin
    b. Towels, warm water, a basin, and soap
    c. Towels, wash cloths, a basin, soap and warm water
    d. Towels, a warm blanket, wash cloths, a basin, soap and warm water

16. You are going to bathe John. The MOST appropriate thing that you should do is

    a. Provide for privacy

    b. Gather your supplies after making certain there is no one in the room but John

    c. Gather your supplies and then provide for John's privacy

    d. Bathe John as long as only family members are present

17. Bath water should be

    a. Changed if it cools

    b. Hot

    c. Soapy

    d. Changed between bathing of each body quadrant

18. You have prepared to bathe John. You are now washing his arms. You should

    a. Use slow circular strokes.

    b. Wash the arm proximal to distal

    c. Wash the arm distal to proximal

    d. Use short strokes away from the heart

19. The taking of John's vital signs includes

    a. Temperature, blood pressure, respirations. and pulse

    b. blood pressure, respirations, pulse and ROM

    c. temperature, I&O, respirations, pulse and blood pressure

    d. All of the above

20. When taking John's blood pressure, you should make certain that

    a.   The cuff is the correct size
    b.   John is lying on his left side
    c.   The cuff is positioned dependent to his elbow
    d.   The cuff is pumped to at least 20 mm above his baseline b/p

21. You will get the most accurate temperature

    a.   Under the arm
    b.   Rectally
    c.   At the groin
    d.   In the ear

22. When counting the pulse rate, what points should you use?

    a.   The carotid artery
    b.   The radial artery
    c.   The apical area of the heart via the chest using a stethoscope
    d.   All of the above

23. While assessing John's temperature, you note that it is 101.2 degrees. What is your FIRST action?

    a.   Notify your supervisor
    b.   Call the doctor
    c.   Wait the appropriate amount of time and take the temperature again
    d.   Have a co-worker check your work.

24. In order that John may be placed in the sitting position in bed, you should first

    a. Check with the charge nurse to make sure the doctor allows that position
    b. Ask someone to assist you in re-positioning him
    c. Clear the patient's room
    d. Take the patient's vital signs

25. You have gotten a co-worker to assist you in repositioning John to a sitting position in bed. Your next action should be to

    a. Lower the bed to a comfortable working height for both you and your assistant
    b. Grasp the draw sheet and count to 3, then lift/pull in the direction of the head of the bed
    c. Explain to John what you are going to do
    d. None of the above

26. You have gotten a co-worker to assist you in re-positioning John and you have explained to him what you are going to do. What is your next action?

    a. Lower the bed to a comfortable working height
    b. Reiterate to John what you will be doing
    c. Assess John's ability to assist you
    d. Grasp the draw sheet, count to 3, then lift/pull toward the top of the bed

27. John is preparing get up out of bed into a wheelchair for the first time after his admission. It is important to encourage him to sit on the side of the bed and dangle his feet for a while to ensure that

    a. Drops his blood pressure.
    b. Has enough will to get up out of bed
    c. Gets dizzy.
    d. He can tolerate the movement.

28. Should you decide to transport John by wheelchair, It is important to remember that you should push him from behind in all of the following scenarios except

    a. entering the elevator
    b. re-entering his room
    c. when you go into the cafeteria
    d. when you are going down the hall

29. When preparing to transfer John from his bed to the wheelchair you should

    a. position the chair at a 45 degree angle at his bedside
    b. position the chair at a 30 degree angle at his bedside and lock the wheels
    c. position the chair to a 45 degree angle at his bedside and lock the wheels
    d. position the chair at a 30 degree angle at his bedside

30. When transferring John to the wheelchair you should make certain that

    a. The wheelchair is sturdy
    b. You have the chair positioned at a 43 degree angle to the bed
    c. Most of the wheels are locked
    d. The bed is in its lowest position

31. When lifting, transferring or moving patients to a chair, the MOST important consideration is

    a.   Comfort
    b.   Documentation
    c.   Protocol
    d.   Safety

Case 2

Paul, a 45-year-old construction worker has been admitted to the hospital for surgery. The doctor has determined that he requires an ostomy. He has been assigned to you for care.

32. When providing ostomy care, you should

    a.   Clean the area around the stoma or ostomy site thoroughly with warm soap and water
    b.   Avoid the ostomy area and clean all surrounding areas thoroughly
    c.   Obtain assistance in cleaning the ostomy area
    d.   Avoid the use of soap on the ostomy area

33. An ostomy site is

    a.   An opening allowing for the exit of urine from the body
    b.   An opening allowing for the exit of stool from the body
    c.   An operative site which has been closed recently requiring frequent dressing changes
    d.   Both a and b

Case 3

Joyce is a 57 year old patient who has been assigned to you. She had surgery yesterday.

34. Joyce begins talking about the death of her sister to you. You should

    a.   Listen
    b.   Leave the room
    c.   Tell her about the death of your brother
    d.   Advise her to talk to her doctor

35. It is appropriate for you to share the information regarding a Joyce's status with

    a.   Any one the nurse aide sees fit
    b.   The client's family members
    c.   The client's roommate
    d.   The staff on the next shift

36. Joyce has developed redness and skin breakdown under her right wrist restraint. If you do not report this occurrence and report it, you are guilty of

    a.   Negligence
    b.   Slander
    c.   Assault
    d.   Threatening a patient

37. On entering Joyce's room, you note that a laboratory technician is attempting to perform to draw blood. He is holding Joyce's arm down forcibly while she is trying to pull away and is calling for help. The tech is guilty of

    a.   Slander
    b.   Assault
    c.   Nothing
    d.   None of the above

38. Joyce requires the use of the bedpan. You should

   a. Turn her on her side with knees flexed
   b. Ask him to lift her hips and place the bedpan beneath his buttocks
   c. Raise her head to a 30 degree angle
   d. None of the above

39. After Joyce has used the bedpan, you should

   a. Empty and rinse the bedpan and store it appropriately
   b. Clean her skin with disposable wipes and dry it
   c. Both a and b
   d. None of the above

40. The doctor has ordered an enema for Joyce. Which of the following do you need to assemble?

   a. Bedpan, incontinence pads, gloves, a pre-prepared enema solution or hospital approved enema equipment, and lubricating solution
   b. Warm water, pads, a bedpan, gloves and an apron
   c. The enema solution, lubricating jell, and incontinence pads
   d. Just the enema solution

41. You should position Joyce

   a. Supine
   b. Lying on her right side
   c. Lying on her left side
   d. Lying on her stomach

42. The Kubler-Ross stages of grief include

   a. Denial, anger and bargaining
   b. Acceptance, bargaining and denial
   c. Depression, anger, acceptance, crying and denial
   d. Denial, anger, bargaining, depression and acceptance

43. Which of the following behavior is not a sign or a symptom of anxiety?

    a. Frequent hand movement
    b. Somatization
    c. The client asks a question
    d. The client is acting out

44. Joyce is angry because of the addition of restraints. What skill would you use to deal with her angry outbursts?

    a. Listening
    b. Advising
    c. Restating
    d. None of the above

45. While dealing with Joyce's bouts of anger, she becomes belligerent and her language toward you is abusive. The proper manner in which to deal with her behavior is

    a. To remain calm
    b. Walk out of the room and tell your co-worker what has occurred so that you can't be sued
    c. Advise Joyce that her behavior is not acceptable
    d. Both a and c

46. A person who is _____ may indicate the desire to place an unconscious barrier between themselves and others.

    a. Avoiding eye contact
    b. Yawning widely
    c. Making wild gestures
    d. Crossing their arms across their chest

47. When communicating with another person, _____ is/are used to emphasize an important point, _____ can show either great interest or boredom, and _____ can express encouragement or empathy.

a. When communicating with another person, gestures are used to emphasize an important point, posture can show either great interest or boredom, and touch can express encouragement or empathy.

b. When communicating with another person, touch is used to emphasize an important point, posture can show either great interest or boredom, and gestures can express encouragement or empathy.

c. When communicating with another person, posture is used to emphasize an important point, gestures can show either great interest or boredom, and touch can express encouragement or empathy.

d. When communicating with another person, gestures are used to emphasize an important point, touch can show either great interest or boredom, and posture can express encouragement or empathy.

48. Which, if any, of the following statements about eye contact are false?

a. Consistent eye contact can indicate a positive reaction to a speaker.

b. Consistent eye contact can indicate a lack of trust in the speaker.

c. The use of eye contact may be dependent on the culture of the listener.

d. None of these statements are false.

49. _____ is a technique used to put people at ease.

   a. Speaking softly
   b. Making eye contact
   c. Mirroring body language
   d. Leaning forward

50. Which, if any, of these statements about body language are false?

   a. Everyone uses some form of body language to communicate.
   b. Interpretations of body language are universal to all cultures.
   c. The study of body language is called kinetic interpretation.
   d. Indications of emotion such as smiling when happy are universal.

51. _____ can signal a lack of interest or an unfriendly attitude and can make therapeutic communication difficult to achieve.

   a. Eye contact
   b. Questioning
   c. Empathy
   d. Nonverbal communication

52. If a patient asks a question that is beyond the scope of your practice, the best response would be to:

   a. Make your best guess based on what you know.
   b. Tell the patient that you will find them the correct answer.
   c. Change the subject.
   d. Give them a book on the subject.

53. What is the recommended method of turning off a hand faucet after washing your hands?

    a. After applying lotion
    a. With a paper or cloth towel
    b. After putting on surgical gloves
    c. None of the Above

54. The most important standard precaution is

    a. Treat all bodily fluids as contaminated
    b. Wear gloves as much as possible
    c. Only wear gloves when you think a patient is contaminated
    d. Always label specimens immediately

55. What federal agency develops and monitors standards for workplace health and safety?

    a. FDA
    b. ADA
    c. OSHA
    d. None of the Above

56. Influenza is caused by

    a. A fungus
    b. Bacteria
    c. A virus
    d. Protozoa

57. A (n) _____ _____ is a legal document filed in advance by a patient which details their wishes if they are incapacitated.

    a. Last will and testament
    b. Beneficiary list
    c. Advance directive
    d. Funeral plan

58. Which if any of the following statements about living wills is true?

    a. They state the type of care a patient does or does not want to receive at the end of their life.

    b. They are documents in which the patient chooses a surrogate who can make healthcare decisions if they are incapacitated.

    c. They demand that no extraordinary measures such as CPR, are used in an effort to revive the patient.

    d. All of the above.

59. What are the two types of advance directives?

    a. A durable power of attorney and a DNR order

    b. A funeral plan and a living will

    c. A life insurance policy and a durable power of attorney

    d. A living will and a durable power of attorney

60. Maintaining _____ requires that information about a patient's current medical status, treatments and discussion of further treatment is only used for its intended purpose.

    a. Confidentiality

    b. Privacy

    c. Discretion

    d. Autonomy

Quick Reference Answer Key

1. B
2. D
3. C
4. A
5. D
6. B
7. C
8. D
9. A
10. B
11. C
12. A
13. A
14. A
15. D
16. C
17. A
18. C
19. A
20. A
21. B
22. D
23. C
24. B
25. C
26. C
27. D
28. A
29. C
30. D
31. D
32. A
33. D
34. A
35. D
36. A
37. B
38. A
39. C
40. A
41. C
42. D
43. C
44. A
45. C
46. D
47. A
48. D
49. C
50. C
51. D
52. B
53. B
54. A
55. C
56. C
57. C
58. D
59. D
60. A

Answer Key with Explanations

1. B
You should always make certain a patient can be shaved and what type of razor is appropriate. If a patient is septic, it may be dangerous for the patient if you shave him at all. Shaving risks a cut that could cause issues with his already compromised immune system.

2. D
You should always shave in the direction of hair growth which changes depending on where you are shaving. Pulling the shin taut allows shaving with minimal risk of cutting.

3. C
The only person who can trim a diabetics nails is a doctor due to potential for infection.

4. A
The appropriate sequence when administering mouth care to a person with dentures is to clean the dentures first. Then you should perform oral care or cleaning. The dentures are then clean and ready for the patient when you have completed oral care.

5. D
Oral care is an essential part of appropriate nursing care. You should give oral care frequently during the day to maintain good oral health.

6. B
You always need gloves when removing dirty linens or performing other tasks which could bring your skin into contact with pathogens or body fluids. Clean linens and a bag for dirty laundry are essential.

7. C
The gloves are removed in such a manner that your skin does not come into contact with contaminated areas of the

gloves and they are turned so that one is contained within the other and appropriately disposed of.

8. D
Unoccupied beds are always made up while in the flat position. Doing so ensures a nice smooth bed which will not irritate the skin. Additionally, it is easier to work with a bed in the flat position than with the head or foot raised.

9. A
You should always observe good body mechanics when working. Raising the bed to a comfortable working height ensures less back strain.

10. B
Dirty linens are always rolled toward the center, keeping any contaminants contained, and placed in the dirty linen bag.

11. C
Part of your duties when making a bed, whether occupied or unoccupied is to make certain that everything, including the mattress, is clean.

12. A
The patient's belongings should always be left in the room where they can easily be located by the patient.

13. A
It is safer for John and will promote more efficient care if you have assistance. Shifting John for changing linens can be difficult physically for one person if the patient is unable to assist you.

14. A
A patient should be bathed daily and then cleaned as needed between each bath.

15. D
You will need clean towels, soap and water and a basin of course. You will also need a blanket to cover John for privacy and dignity and to provide warmth while you bathe him.

16. C
John is entitled to privacy while receiving a bath. Family members are no exception. If you wait until after you provide for privacy to gather your equipment, it may be necessary to empty the room again of visitors.

17. A
Water should be maintained at a comfortable temperature for bathing. It should always be changed and replaced with warm water if it cools.

18. C
Hands and arms are always washed distal to proximal. You should always wash from cleanest to dirtiest. The armpit is considered dirty. In addition, you should always wash the patient using strokes that lead toward the heart. This increases venous return.

19. A
The four components of the vital sign assessment are temperature, blood pressure, pulse, and respirations.

20. A
If the cuff is not the proper width for your patient, you will get a false reading on your blood pressure check.

21. B
The rectal temperature is taken within the body cavity and therefore yields a temperature reading closest to actual body temperature.

22. D
The pulse can accurately be counted using any of these areas, although for most initial assessments the radial pulse is used.

23. C
Always double-check your vital signs to make certain there is a valid problem.

24. B
When repositioning a patient, it is always in the best interest of the patient and the nurse to obtain assistance. This

allows for safety for both.

25. C
Never attempt to perform an action for the patient without first explaining what you are going to do and how you will be going about it.

26. C
The MOST appropriate answer is c. You should always allow the patient to do whatever they can to assist in their own care. Never exclude them!

27. D
Many things occur within the body when position is changed; blood pressure may rise or fall. The patient is most likely already weakened from having been bed bound. While the patient is sitting bedside, you can evaluate his ability to move safely.

28. A
A wheelchair bound patient is always turned facing outward and backed into an elevator. This prevents disorientation and dizziness on the part of the patient as well as promoting the use of good body mechanics for the nurse.

29. C
A 45-degree angle allows space to assist your patient in the transfer but not so much that you can't stabilize him is he slips. A 30-degree angle would be too wide to allow for control over a fall. Wheelchair wheels are ALWAYS locked.

30. D
The bed must be in the lowest position possible for both the safety of the patient as well as the nurse. Try to get the area we are transferring the patient from as close as possible. This will enable us to 'pivot' with John rather than manually carry him to his wheelchair.

31. D
The safety of both patient and nurse is foremost in the transferring of patients.

32. A
The skin surrounding the ostomy site must be kept clean and dry. Enzymes from exudate can erode the skin if proper care is not implemented.

33. D
An ostomy is used to allow for the exit of feces and urine when a patient's body can no longer perform this function normally.

34. A
You need to listen when your patient begins to talk about loss. It is part of your therapeutic intervention as a professional.

35. D
Staff members involved with your patient's care are the only ones you can share information. Giving report to the next shift is appropriate.

36. A
If you do not address the change in status of a patient, but rather ignore it, you are guilty of professional negligence and can be held accountable.

37. B
Assault is the unauthorized or forcible touching of another person.

38. A
When preparing to place a patient on the bedpan, you should have him/her positioned on one side with knees flexed, place the bedpan beneath the buttocks and have them roll over onto the bedpan using their flexed knees to lift their hips and position themselves comfortably on the bedpan.

39. C
Skin care is always provided after bedpan use to prevent tissue breakdown. You must always empty and rinse the bedpan and store it appropriately after use.

40. A
You would need all this equipment to perform the enema, protect yourself and the patient's linens and to lubricate the anal opening for ease of entry.

41. C
The patient is positioned on the left side to facilitate entry of the enema fluid into the colon. The colon is situated within the abdomen such that the flow of the enema fluid from this position would enter the rectum flowing naturally into the descending colon and on across the transverse colon to the ascending colon.

42. D
The five phases of this grief model include denial, anger, bargaining, depression and acceptance.

43. C
If the client is asking questions, they are coping with feelings. All of the other answers are symptoms of an anxious patient.

44. A
To address the reason for her anger, you must listen to why she is angry.

45. C
It is appropriate to advise a patient that abusive behavior is unacceptable. Above all, you MUST remain calm and professional.

46. D
A person who is **crossing their arms across their chest** may indicate the desire to place an unconscious barrier between themselves and others.

47. A
When communicating with another person, gestures are used to emphasize an important point, posture can indicate either great interest or boredom, and touch can express encouragement or empathy.

48. D
None of these statements are false.
Consistent eye contact can indicate a positive reaction to a speaker.

Consistent eye contact can indicate a lack of trust in the speaker.

The use of eye contact may depend on the culture of the listener.

49. C
The idea of mirroring body language to put people at ease is commonly used in interviews. Mirroring the body language shows that they are understood.

50. C
The study of body language is called kinetic interpretation is false.

51. D
Nonverbal communication can signal a lack of interest or an unfriendly attitude, and can make therapeutic communication difficult to achieve.

52. B
If a patient asks a question and you do not know the answer, the best response is the response that is the most helpful. I.e. that you will help this in finding the answer. Saying that you don't know or similar responses are not helpful to the patient.

53. B
Turning off the tap with a paper towel prevents contamination from the tap.

54. A
The most important standard precaution is **to treat all bodily fluids as contaminated.**

55. C
The United States Occupational Safety and Health Administration (OSHA) is an agency of the United States Department of Labor. Its mission is to prevent work-related in-

juries, illnesses, and occupational fatality by issuing and enforcing standards for workplace safety and health.

56. C

Influenza, commonly referred to as the flu, is an infectious disease caused by RNA viruses of the family Orthomyxoviridae (the influenza viruses), that affects birds and mammals. The most common symptoms of the disease are chills, fever, sore throat, muscle pains, severe headache, coughing, weakness/fatigue and general discomfort. Although it is often confused with other influenza-like illnesses, especially the common cold, influenza is a more severe disease than the common cold and is caused by a different type of virus.[1]

57. C

An **advance directive** is a legal document filed in advance by a patient which details their wishes if they are incapacitated.

An advance health care directive, also known as living will, personal directive, advance directive, or advance decision, are instructions given by individuals specifying what actions should be taken for their health if they are no longer able to make decisions due to illness or incapacity, and appoints a person to make such decisions on their behalf. A living will is one form of advance directive, leaving instructions for treatment. Another form authorizes a specific type of power of attorney or health care proxy, where someone is appointed by the individual to make decisions on their behalf when they are incapacitated. People may also have a combination of both. It is often encouraged that people complete both documents to provide the most comprehensive guidance regarding their care. One example of a combination document is the Five Wishes advance directive in the United States.[2]

58. D

The following are true about living wills:

They are documents in which the patient chooses a surrogate who can make healthcare decisions if they are incapacitated.

They demand that no extraordinary measures such as CPR, are used in an effort to revive the patient.

59. D
Two types of advance directives are **a living will and a durable power of attorney.**

An advance health care directive, also known as living will, personal directive, advance directive, or advance decision, are instructions given by individuals specifying what actions should be taken for their health if they are no longer able to make decisions due to illness or incapacity, and appoints a person to make such decisions on their behalf. A living will is one form of advance directive, leaving instructions for treatment. Another form authorizes a specific type of power of attorney or health care proxy, where the individual appoints someone to make decisions on their behalf when they are incapacitated. People may also have a combination of both. It is often encouraged that people complete both documents to provide the most comprehensive guidance regarding their care. One example of a combination document is the Five Wishes advance directive in the United States.[2]

60. A
Maintaining confidentiality requires that information about a patient's current medical status, treatments and discussion of further treatment is only used for its intended purpose.

Practice Test 2

The practice test presents questions representative of questions you can expect to find on the NNAAP. However, they are not intended to match exactly what is on the NNAAP.

For the best results, take this Practice Test as if it were the real exam. Set aside time when you will not be disturbed, and a location that is quiet and free of distractions. Read the instructions carefully, read each question carefully, and answer to the best of your ability.

Use the bubble answer sheets provided. When you have completed the Practice Test, check your answer against the Answer Key and read the explanation provided.

Answer Sheet – Practice Test II

	A	B	C	D	E			A	B	C	D	E
1	○	○	○	○	○		26	○	○	○	○	○
2	○	○	○	○	○		27	○	○	○	○	○
3	○	○	○	○	○		28	○	○	○	○	○
4	○	○	○	○	○		29	○	○	○	○	○
5	○	○	○	○	○		30	○	○	○	○	○
6	○	○	○	○	○		31	○	○	○	○	○
7	○	○	○	○	○		32	○	○	○	○	○
8	○	○	○	○	○		33	○	○	○	○	○
9	○	○	○	○	○		34	○	○	○	○	○
10	○	○	○	○	○		35	○	○	○	○	○
11	○	○	○	○	○		36	○	○	○	○	○
12	○	○	○	○	○		37	○	○	○	○	○
13	○	○	○	○	○		38	○	○	○	○	○
14	○	○	○	○	○		39	○	○	○	○	○
15	○	○	○	○	○		40	○	○	○	○	○
16	○	○	○	○	○		41	○	○	○	○	○
17	○	○	○	○	○		42	○	○	○	○	○
18	○	○	○	○	○		43	○	○	○	○	○
19	○	○	○	○	○		44	○	○	○	○	○
20	○	○	○	○	○		45	○	○	○	○	○
21	○	○	○	○	○		46	○	○	○	○	○
22	○	○	○	○	○		47	○	○	○	○	○
23	○	○	○	○	○		48	○	○	○	○	○
24	○	○	○	○	○		49	○	○	○	○	○
25	○	○	○	○	○		50	○	○	○	○	○

1. When performing a patient's oral care, you should first

    a. Place his head at a 45 degree angle
    b. Place his head flat and have him turn his head to one side
    c. Have him swish his mouth with mouthwash
    d. Clean inside his mouth using gentle circular motions

2. Patient's oral care should include

    a. Denture care
    b. Gentle cleaning of the oral mucosa and lips
    c. Cleaning of the tongue
    d. All of the above

3. Your co-worker tells you that the doctor has ordered cold packs for a patient's sprained wrist. You are aware that

    a. You should assess their skin before applying the pack and document your findings
    b. The cold pack should be applied for no longer than twenty minutes per interval
    c. You should read the order thoroughly prior to administering the cold pack.
    d. All of the above

4. After applying a cold pack, you should reassess the patient's skin

    a. Every 5 minutes
    b. Every 10 minutes
    c. As often as you can
    d. Only after the 20 minute treatment has been completed

5. After application of the cold pack you should

   a. Document that the order was carried out, the skin condition before and after application and the duration of the treatment

   b. Document that the order was carried out and sign the chart

   c. Remove the cold pack and properly dispose of it and tell your co-worker that you have completed the treatment

   d. All of the above

6. Your co-worker has rolled John onto his right side. The top sheet has been removed. To remove the bottom layers and replace them you would

   a. Roll the dirty linen from the edge of the bed inward toward John.

   b. Roll the dirty linen from the top toward John's waist making certain that the dirty side is rolled toward the center then roll the remaining linen from John's feet toward the center taking the same care to keep the dirty side toward the center

   c. Pull the dirty linen out from under John's body and place it in the dirty linen bag

   d. Place the clean linen on top of the soiled linen and then remove the dirty linen appropriately placing in the dirty linen container

7. Should you determine that John can help you safely, when preparing to change John's linens you would

   a. Lower the bedrail on the side opposite you leaving the other rail raised while working

   b. Lower the bedrail closest to you leaving the other rail raised while working

   c. Lower both bedrails while working

   d. Lower the bed to its lowest position before beginning

8. It is necessary to keep John covered while you are making his bed

   a. Only if there are others in the room
   b. Always
   c. If the room is cool
   d. Until you get the draw sheet in place

9. When making John's bed, you have replaced the bottom linens on your side. Your coworker is preparing to complete the change of linens. You assist John in rolling over. Your co-worker would then

   a. Grasp the roll of clean linens and unroll them from center toward the side of the bed making certain they were smooth and wrinkle free
   b. Grasp the linens and pull hard so that the linens will be wrinkle free
   c. Raise the bed rail
   d. Place clean linens under John making certain they were wrinkle free.

10. After you have completed making John's bed, you should wash your hands. The proper manner in which you would do this is

   a. Wash your hands using plenty of warm water and soap, thoroughly rinse and dry
   b. Wash your hands, including cleaning your nails, using plenty of warm soap and water, rinse and dry
   c. Wash your hands, including nails, using warm water and soap, rinse and dry
   d. Wash your hands and clean your nails using warm water and soap, rinse and dry using your towel to turn off the water

11. You should wash your hands

   a. 4 times daily
   b. Before and after patient contact
   c. When they become soiled
   d. Both b and c

12. You have placed a patient in a semi-sitting position. The head of his bed is at 45 degrees. This position is called

   a. Recumbent
   b. Flexed
   c. Sim's
   d. Fowler's

13. A patient is lying on his side with his thigh flexed. The doctor is preparing to perform a rectal examination. This position is appropriately named

   a. Fowler's
   b. Freud's
   c. Sim's
   d. Sam's

14. When bathing a patient, you should

   a. ALWAYS use soap, clean towels and warm water
   b. Use firms strokes in the direction of the heart
   c. Rub briskly with your cloth to stimulate circulation
   d. Wait until later in your day because it will take a long time to bathe him

15. When dressing a patient you should always

    a.   Let him do what he can on his own and assist with what he can't do

    b.   Do everything for him

    c.   Insist that he dress himself because it is therapeutic for him to be independent

    d.   Get someone to assist you

16. You have completed a patient's bath and are preparing to dress him. You have provided a clean shirt. The patient has weakness on the left side from a stoke. To put his shirt on, which arm should you put into the sleeve first?

    a.   Both

    b.   Left

    c.   Right

    d.   Let John choose

17. A back massage is

    a.   Not a part of the bathing duties

    b.   The time when skin assessment can be made

    c.   Included in bathing

    d.   Both b and c

18. Bathing is performed to

    a.   Remove bacteria from the skin surface

    b.   Promote relaxation

    c.   Improve circulation

    d.   All of the above

19. You are going to transfer a patient from his bed to a chair. You have placed the chair at the appropriate angle and the bed is in lowest potion. Which of the following is the BEST way to complete the transfer?

   a. Using your back and arms, pull John upright and pivot toward the chair and gently settle him into the chair
   b. Wrapping your arms around John's torso and with knees slightly bent; use your legs to turn with the patient. Ask the patient, if he is capable, to grasp the arm of the chair. If now, slowly back toward the chair until you feel with your own leg that it is there. Slowly lower John into the chair.
   c. Using only your arms and legs, lift the patient into your arms and settle him safely into his chair.
   d. Obtain assistance from a co-worker. Each of you take one side of the patient and gently lift, using proper body mechanics, and transfer him to his chair.

20. What is the rationale for getting a patient out of bed?

   a. To maintain muscle tone
   b. To improve muscle tone
   c. To allow for adequate pulmonary function
   d. All of the above

21. Which of the following is NOT a stage of assisting a patient in getting out of bed safely?

   a. Assist the patient to stand
   b. Allow John to dangle his feet over the side of the bed
   c. Assist John in moving to the chair
   d. Asking a family member to explain to John what you are about to do

22. Which would you do first when assisting a patient out of bed?

    a. Assist him to a standing position

    b. Allow him to dangle his feet over the edge of the bed

    c. Move the chair out of his way

    d. Obtain the chair from across the room

23. A patient is being transferred to a chair. You and a co-worker are helping him. Which part of your anatomy should be MOST involved in the transfer?

    a. Legs
    b. Back
    c. Arms and shoulders
    d. Both b and c

24. If the patient begins to become off balance or unstable during the transfer, you should

    a. Attempt to stabilize the patient by bracing him against you and guide the patient to the bedside or chair, if possible.

    b. If a fall begins to occur, guide him slowly toward the floor.

    c. Move back and allow the patient to slide to the floor and call for assistance

    d. Both a and b

25. If a fall occurs, as you gently glide your patient to the floor you should

    a. Protect his head
    b. Protect his IV
    c. Protect his drains
    d. Protect his extremities

26. After a patient's fall, the first thing that you should do is

   a. Call for assistance in getting John off the floor and into bed or his chair
   b. Just pick him up and complete the move
   c. Assess for injuries and call for assistance
   d. Talk to your assistant about what went wrong

27. After a patient's fall, what document must you fill out?

   a. And incident report
   b. The I & O sheet
   c. Charting of the people who witnessed the fall
   d. The vital sign flow sheet

28. While walking by a co-worker, you overhear her telling another worker that you have not addressed a patient's restraint care in your documentation. You are aware that this is untrue and that you have done all that you should do for your patient. Your co-worker's behavior is an example of

   a. Slander
   b. Assault
   c. Defamation
   d. Both a and d

29. After coming on duty later in the course of a patient's care, you note that her restraints have been tied to the bed frame. You are aware that this can cause injury to the patient and is inappropriate use of her restraints. This is an example of

   a. Assault
   b. Negligence
   c. Appropriate action
   d. Slander

30. You have just walked into a patient's room and you overhear a lab technician telling her to allow him to draw her blood or he will tighten her restraints. The lab tech is guilty of

   a. Slander
   b. Threatening a patient
   c. Acting in the patient's best interest
   d. Violation of Joyce's privacy

31. Restraints may be used

   a. To force her to obey doctor's orders no matter what
   b. Only at night
   c. In accordance with doctor's orders only
   d. None of the above

32. All of the following are inappropriate within the scope of the hospital setting EXCEPT

   a. Documentation
   b. Providing for patient privacy
   c. Talking about a co-worker
   d. Using gloves

33. A patient has become confused and her doctor has ordered wrist restraints. All the following are true of restraints except

   a. They should allow as much freedom of movement as possible
   b. They should be removed periodically
   c. Their application should be documented
   d. They should be tied to the bed frame

34. The patient has attempted to get out of bed and has managed to slip despite her wrist restraints. The doctor orders the addition of ankle restraints. You know that

   a. The use of restraints on all four extremities is also termed 'four point restraints'
   b. Range of motion exercises should be performed regularly
   c. You should observe for skin breakdown
   d. All of the above

35. Prior to application of the patient's ankle restraints, she kicked the side rail bruising her knee and causing minor swelling. The doctor has ordered that a cold pack be applied to the area. You would know that

   a. The cold pack will help with swelling and pain as well as bruising
   b. You should leave the cold pack in place no longer than 20 minutes
   c. You should assess the skin prior to applying the cold pack
   d. All of the above

36. Before you apply the patient's cold pack, you assess her skin integrity, temperature and color. You note that the skin is extremely cold, blue-black in color in an area extending beyond the damaged originally damaged area, the tissue is extremely swollen and Joyce is complaining of intense pain. You should

   a. Not apply the cold pack until you have reported your findings to the charge nurse or doctor
   b. Go ahead and apply the cold pack
   c. Initiate a CODE BLUE
   d. Gently massage the area before applying the cold pack

37. While assessing John's temperature, you note that it is 101.2 degrees. What is your FIRST action?

    a. Notify your supervisor
    b. Call the doctor
    c. Wait the appropriate amount of time and take the temperature again
    d. Have a co-worker check your work.

38. You can count respirations while

    a. Taking John's b/p
    b. Counting John's pulse
    c. Taking his temperature
    d. None of the above

39. When assessing a patient's respirations you should

    a. Count the number of times his chest rises and falls in one minute
    b. Auscultate his chest
    c. Observe whether John is breathing easily or seems to be having difficulty
    d. All of the above

40. If a patient's 3 year old granddaughter was visiting and was watching you take her grandfather's vital signs and became curious about how you would take hers, you might explain to her that

    a. You would do it on the arm but with a smaller cuff
    b. You would do it on her thigh but with a smaller cuff
    c. You would do it on her ankle using a smaller cuff
    d. All of the above.

41. You came on duty at 7 A.M. It is now 1 P.M. Assuming everything is normal, how many times should you have assessed John's vital sign status?

   a. Twice
   b. Once
   c. PRN
   d. Not at all

42. After assessing a patient's vitals, the MOST proper way to document them would be

   a. Bp140/72, Pulse regular and bounding, Respirations 16 and shallow, temp. 99.0
   b. Temp 99.0 orally, BP 140/72, Pulse regular, Respirations 16
   c. Pulse regular and bounding, Temp. 99.0 orally, B/P140/72, Respirations 16 and shallow
   d. None of the above

43. When taking a rectal temperature you will need

   a. Gloves and lubricant
   b. An oral thermometer
   c. A rectal thermometer
   d. Both a and c

Case 3

Joyce is a 57 year old patient who has been assigned to you. She had surgery yesterday. She has mentioned the loss of a family member to you several times.

44. In reviewing the care that you have administered to Joyce today, you are aware that her anger may have been

   a. A stage of grief
   b. Caused by her dislike of you
   c. Caused by a hereditary disease
   d. Temporary insanity

45. To assist Joyce in accepting the loss of her family member you must

   a. Read everything on death and dying before approaching her
   b. Be willing to talk with her about death
   c. Not bring up her loss, no matter what
   d. Distract her with conversation about other things

46. James, a 19-year-old college student has been admitted to the hospital for sports injuries sustained during a hockey game. He has been assigned to you. When you enter his room to take him his breakfast tray, he comments on your appearance and tries to touch you. You should

   a. Tell him that his actions are inappropriate
   b. Ignore him
   c. Slap his hand
   d. Call for help

47. After telling James that his actions are inappropriate, he apologizes and you leave the room. You should

   a. Document the occurrence and your response
   b. Call the police
   c. Talk to your co-workers to obtain support
   d. Ignore the incident

48. Joyce's family has been in to visit her. They have told her that her sister was killed in an automobile accident. While performing her care, you note that she is silent and withdrawn. You would know that this she is experiencing which of the Kubler-Ross stages of grief?

   a. Acceptance
   b. Denial
   c. Bargaining
   d. Depression

49. _____ is restating something that a patient has said, usually in fewer words and with emphasis on the main points of their statement.

- a. Attending
- b. Paraphrasing
- c. Clarifying
- d. Perception checking

50. Facial expression, posture and tone of voice are elements of _____.

- a. Open-ended questions
- b. Nonverbal communication
- c. Orientation process
- d. Good manners

51. Which, if any, of the following statements about nonverbal communication are true?

a. Nonverbal communications are less reliable that verbal communication

b. Nonverbal communications remain the same, regardless of ethnicity or culture.

c. Nonverbal communications always send a clear message.

d. Nonverbal communications can emphasize or contradict verbal messages.

52. _____ provides encourages the patient to continue talking without showing agreement or disagreement.

- a. Smiling
- b. Leaning forward
- c. Nodding
- d. Paraphrasing

53. Using phrases that address a person's feelings, such as "You must be worried about your headaches," demonstrates _____.

    a. Empathy
    b. Interest
    c. Acceptance
    d. Recognition

54. When dealing with elderly patients, always _____.

    a. Use their first names to establish intimacy.
    b. Direct your questions to their caregivers.
    c. Speak loudly and distinctly.
    d. Address them as Miss, Mrs., or Mr., followed by their last name.

55. When interviewing a patient with a hearing loss, remember to _____.

    a. Speak slowly and look directly at the patient.
    b. Ensure that the room is brightly lit.
    c. Write down your questions and have them write their answers.
    d. Both a) and b).

56. A/an _____ is a form that is filled out as soon as possible following an event such as an injury to a patient.

    a. Tort
    b. Occurrence statement
    c. Testimonial
    d. Incident report

57. Using neutral remarks such as, "I see" and "I hear what you're saying" show _____ to the patient.

    a. Empathy
    b. Recognition
    c. Understanding
    d. Avoidance

58. If a patient refuses to make eye contact, you may find that they are _____.

    a. From a culture that considers direct eye contact rude.
    b. Very tired.
    c. Lying about their symptoms.
    d. Disinterested in the conversation.

59. When communicating with non-English speaking patients, professionals should:

    a. Repeat sentences word-for-word if the patient does not understand.
    b. Use their children as interpreters.
    c. Raise the volume of their voices.
    d. Immediately employ the services of an interpreter.

60. Which, if any, of the following statements about geriatrics are false?

    a. Geriatrics is a branch of medicine in which the focus is health care for the aging population.
    b. Geriatrics differs from gerontology, which is the study of the aging process itself.
    c. A geriatrician's practice is limited to persons over the age of 65.
    d. None of the above.

Quick Reference Answer Key

1. A
2. D
3. D
4. B
5. A
6. A
7. B
8. B
9. A
10. D
11. D
12. D
13. C
14. B
15. A
16. B
17. D
18. D
19. B
20. D
21. D
22. B
23. A
24. A
25. A
26. C
27. A
28. D
29. B
30. B
31. C
32. C
33. D
34. D
35. D
36. A
37. C
38. C
39. D
40. D
41. A
42. B
43. D
44. A
45. B
46. A
47. A
48. D
49. B
50. B
51. D
52. C
53. A
54. D
55. A
56. D
57. C
58. A
59. D
60. C

Answer Key with Explanations

1. A
Always place the head at this angle to prevent choking.

2. D
Mouth care includes all areas of the mouth both inside and out.

3. D
You never take an order from another person. Always check the chart yourself and read the order. You should assess skin integrity at every opportunity, especially with diabetics. Cold packs are NEVER left in place longer than 20 minutes.

4. B
You should always reassess skin 10 minutes after the application of a cold pack.

5. A
You should always document after a procedure is carried out. Note everything that you can about the area of treatment both before treatment is performed and afterward.

6. A
Always roll dirty linen toward the center to contain contaminates.

7. B
Lowering the rail nearest you allows you to work and leaving the opposite rail raised provide for John's safety by preventing a fall from the bed.

8. B
You should always keep a clean sheet, blanket or bath blanket over the patient even when replacing top linens. This is done to provide for warmth and privacy.

9. A
The linens are already under John, the bedrail should already be down, and you do not pull hard on linens that

a patient is lying on as this could injure the patient.

10. D
You would use the paper towel utilized to dry your hands to turn off the water avoiding contamination of your clean hands.

11. D
Hand washing is a critical part of patient care and personal safety.

12. D
Fowler's positioning is considered to be an upright position of varying degrees.

13. C
Sim's position is a side lying position with the patient's thigh flexed. This position facilitates access to the rectum and vagina for examination.

14. B
You can't always use soap, especially with geriatric patients. You should ALWAYS use strokes that travel in the direction heading toward the heart as this increases venous return.

15. A
Allowing John to do what he can promotes independence and dignity in a difficult situation. Offer assistance when needed.

16. B
When a patient has weakness in an extremity, that extremity is always dressed first.

17. D
A gentle back massage is part of the bathing process and allows inspection of the skin on the back and buttocks as well as documentation and reporting of any adverse findings.

18. D
The removal of bacteria, relaxation and improved circulation are all benefits of bathing.

19. B
None of the other answers take into account the proper use of body mechanics except for answer d. Answer d is incorrect because this exercise involves a one on one move....not an assisted move.

20. D
It is critical, if proper functioning of body systems is to be secured, that movement be encouraged when feasible. Extended time as a bed-bound patient impairs normal system functioning.

21. D
You should be the one explaining what is happening to John.

22. B
You must allow John to dangle his feet over the edge of the bed for a short time. This allows for settling of equilibrium, blood pressure changes to settle, and blood flow to extremities time to alter.

23. A
Carry the majority of the force of the move on your legs. This prevents damage to the nurses back, arms and shoulders. All play a role in the transfer, but carry the bulk of the weight on your legs.

24. A
Should a fall begin to occur, your first priority is to protect the patient. Stabilize him with your body by bracing him against you and if it is impossible to avoid a fall then your only alternative is to guide him, gently to the floor.

25. A
The correct answer is to protect John's head. IV's, drains and extremities are all important, but a head blow could be very serious, even lethal.

26. C
Of course, you will need assistance in getting him off the floor, but your first priority is in ascertaining whether John has sustained injuries due to the fall. You should

NOT move him further without both assistance and assessment.

27. A
Whenever an unexpected occurrence happens which involves a patient, or even a worker, you MUST fill out an incident report.

28. D
Your co-worker has spoken about you to others and the things said were untrue and could damage your reputation and endanger your license.

29. B
Properly trained medical personnel know that a hospital bed is created to move. Tying restraints to the bed will injure a patient at some point when the position of the bed is changed and must be avoided.

30. B
The tech has threatened Joyce with action he is not authorized to perform and which may cause her fear and anxiety to elicit her cooperation. This is inappropriate behavior.

31. C
Forcing a patient to do anything using restraints constitutes abuse and negligence. You must only use restraints in accordance with her doctor's orders.

32. C
Talking about a co-worker can constitute slander and defamation of character. At the least, it is unprofessional conduct and you should avoid.

33. D
A, b, and c are all true of the appropriate use of restraints. Tying the restraint off to the bed frame places the patient in jeopardy if the position of the bed is changed.

34. D
You always perform ROM exercises on restrained limbs regularly and the potential for skin breakdown is in-

creased with the addition of restraints. The term 'four point restraints' is indicative that four extremities have been restrained.

35. D
Cold packs are extremely therapeutic in the treatment of bruising, swelling and pain, however you should continually assess the patient's skin during their use and they should be limited to an application time not to exceed 20 minutes per treatment. The skin should then be reassessed and proper documentation performed.

36. A
For a minor injury, you should not see these symptoms. Blue-black tissue, intense pain and extremely cool skin could indicate a blood clot or more serious tissue damage than was originally thought. You should report your findings to the proper authority.

37. C
Always double-check your vital signs to make certain there is a valid problem.

38. C
While the thermometer is registering John's temperature, it is a good time to count his respirations. This is an example of good time management.

39. D
The respiratory assessment should ALWAYS include the number of respirations, the quality of them and accompanying breath sounds.

40. D
A child of this age could have her b/p assessed on any of the above-mentioned areas using a child's cuff.

41. A
Within the 6 hours you have been on duty, given that you are to assess his vital signs every 4 hours, you should have documented them twice.

42. B
When noting vital signs you must give as much information as you have been able to obtain. This should include the count, quality, and anything abnormal.

43. D
An oral thermometer is never used to take a rectal temperature. Gloves, lubricant and a rectal thermometer are the appropriate implements utilized during this phase of vital signs.

44. A
Anger is one of the stages of grief and Joyce has just experienced the loss of a loved one.

45. B
You must be willing to talk to her about death. At some point, this is something that any patient who experiences a loss will do.

46. A
Setting boundaries for sexual conduct in the workplace is important.

47. A
You should always document harassment of any kind as well as your response. It is your protection. Remember, if you don't document, it NEVER happened.

48. D
Joyce is exhibiting symptoms of withdrawal and silence. She is not talking, actively grieving, or crying.

49. B
Paraphrasing is restating something that a patient has said, usually in fewer words and with emphasis on the main points of their statement.

50. B
Facial expression, posture and tone of voice are elements of nonverbal communication.

51. D
Nonverbal communications can emphasize or contradict verbal messages is the only statement that is true.

52. C
Nodding provides encourages the patient to continue talking without indicating agreement or disagreement.

53. A
Using phrases that address a person's feelings, such as "You must be worried about your headaches," demonstrates empathy.

54. D
Always address older patients Miss, Mrs., or Mr., followed by their last name. Addressing older patients by their first name may offend.

55. A
When interviewing a patient with a hearing loss, remember to speak slowly and look directly at the patient.

56. D
In a health care facility, such as a hospital, nursing home, or assisted living, an incident report or accident report is a form that is filled out to record details of an unusual event that occurs at the facility, such as an injury to a patient. The purpose of the incident report is to document the exact details of the occurrence while they are fresh in the minds of those who witnessed the event. This information may be useful in the future when dealing with liability issues stemming from the incident.

Generally, according to health care guidelines, the report must be filled out when possible following the incident (but after the situation has been stabilized). This way, the details written in the report are as accurate as possible.

Most incident reports that are written involve accidents with patients, such as patient falls. However, most facilities will also document an incident in which a staff member or visitor is injured.

If an incident involves a patient, the patient will often be monitored for a period of time following the incident (for it may happen again), which may include taking vital signs regularly. 3

57. C
Using neutral remarks such as, "I see" and "I hear what you're saying" indicates understanding to the patient.

58. A
If a patient refuses to make eye contact, you may find that they are from a culture that considers direct eye contact rude.

59. D
If the patient has 'no' English at all, which is a little rare but does happen, then using an interpreter is the best choice. If the patient has 'a little' English, then speak slowly and carefully. Raising your voice will not help.

60. C
A geriatrician's practice is limited to persons over the age of 65 is false. Geriatrics is a sub-specialty of internal medicine and family medicine that focuses on health care of elderly people. It aims to promote health by preventing and treating diseases and disabilities in older adults. There is no set age at which patients may be under the care of a geriatrician, or physician who specializes in the care of elderly people. Rather, this decision is determined by the individual patient's needs, and the availability of a specialist.[4]

Conclusion

CONGRATULATIONS! You have made it this far because you have applied yourself diligently to practicing for the exam and no doubt improved your potential score considerably! Getting into a good school is a huge step in a journey that might be challenging at times but will be many times more rewarding and fulfilling. That is why being prepared is so important.

Study then Practice and then Succeed!

Good Luck!

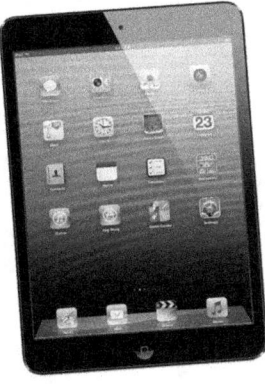

FREE Ebook Version

Download a FREE Ebook version of the publication!

Suitable for tablets, iPad, iPhone, or any smart phone.

Go to
http://tinyurl.com/m5dyb68

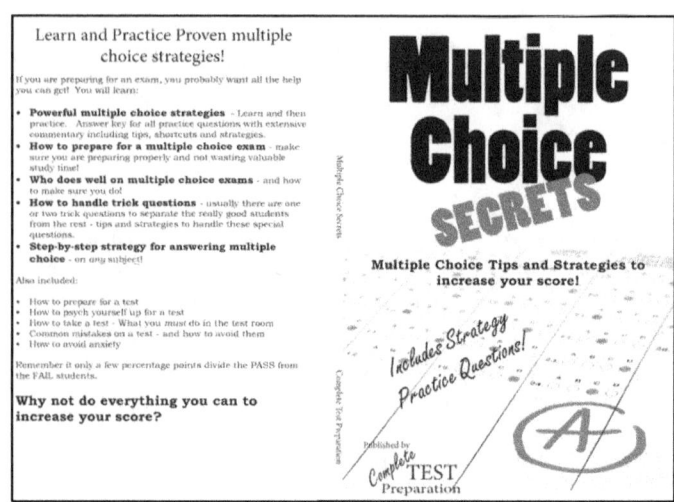

Learn to increase your score using time-tested secrets for answering multiple choice questions!

You will learn 12 strategies for answering multiple choice questions and then practice each strategy with over 45 reading comprehension multiple choice questions, with extensive commentary from exam experts!

Maybe you have read this kind of thing before, and maybe feel you don't need it, and you are not sure if you are going to buy this Book.

Remember though, it only a few percentage points divide the PASS from the FAIL students.

Even if our multiple choice strategies increase your score by a few percentage points, isn't that worth it?

https://www.createspace.com/3889980

Enter Code LYFZGQB5 for 25% off

Thanks!

If you enjoyed this book and would like to order additional copies for yourself or for friends, please check with your local bookstore, favourite online bookseller or visit www.test-preparation.ca and place your order directly with the publisher.

Feedback to the publisher may be sent by email to feedback@test-preparation.ca

www.ingramcontent.com/pod-product-compliance
Lightning Source LLC
LaVergne TN
LVHW010302260326
834688LV00044B/1423